Essential Oils for Weight Loss

Disclaimer and Terms of Use:

Effort has been made to ensure that the information in this book is accurate and complete, however, the author and the publisher do not warrant the accuracy of the information, text and graphics contained within the book due to the rapidly changing nature of science, research, known and unknown facts and internet. The Author and the publisher do not hold any responsibility for errors, omissions or contrary interpretation of the subject matter herein. This book is presented solely for motivational and informational purposes only.

Table of Contents

Introduction

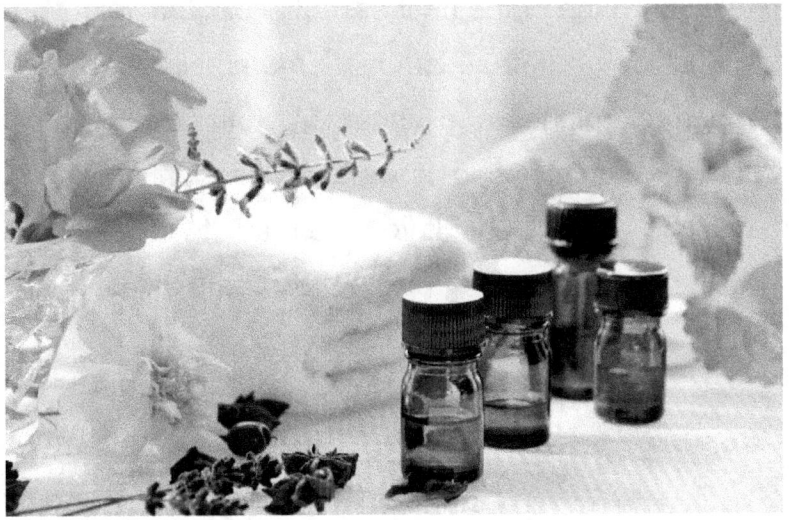

Essential oils are a type of liquid extract that come from different plants – they are named essential oils because they contain the "essence" of the plant from which they are extracted. The essential oil of various plants is the substance that contains the plant's fragrance as well as most of its health benefits. Essential oils can be used for a wide variety of different purposes from aromatherapy, to herbal remedies, even weight loss! Different essential oils have different properties, they do not all provide the same benefits related to weight loss. Some essential oils help to suppress your appetite while others help to reduce the appearance of cellulite or to curb cravings. Some of the best essential oils for weight loss include grapefruit, lemon, bergamot, sandalwood, peppermint, ginger, and cinnamon. In this book, you will receive a collection of twenty-five essential oils recipes for weight loss. If you are ready to kick-start your weight loss efforts, pick a recipe and give it a try!

Essential Oils for Weight Loss Recipes

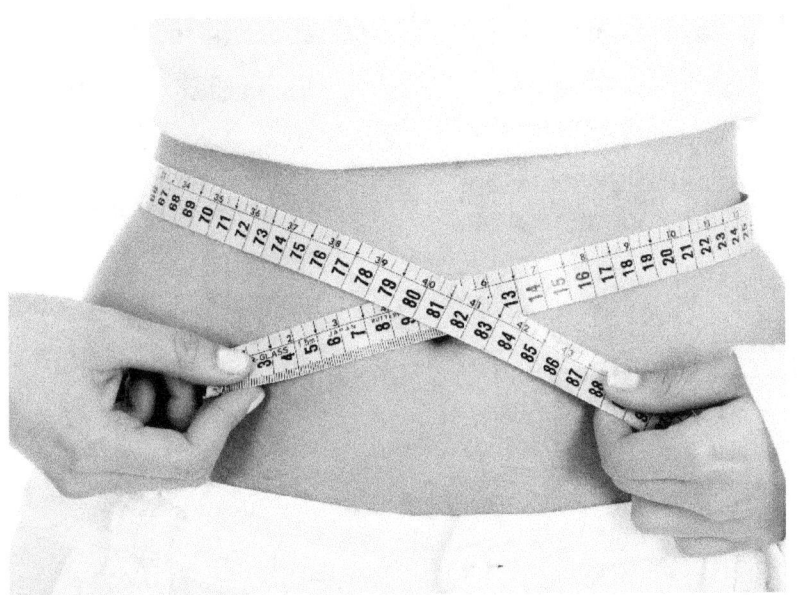

Recipes Included in this Book:

Energy-Boosting Foot Rub

Fat-Blasting Grapefruit Rub

Cinnamon Drink for Fullness

Refreshing, Anti-Stress Bath

Lemon Detox Massage

Pre-Dinner Appetite Suppressant

Soothing Sandalwood Coconut Milk Beverage

Craving-Cutting Inhalation

Uplifting Peppermint Rub

Anti-Bloat Grapefruit Drink

Bergamot Craving Suppressant Inhalation

Appetite-Reducing Grapefruit Inhalation

All-Day Weight Loss Drink

Soothing Detoxification Bath

Appetite-Suppressant Cinnamon Inhalation

Sandalwood Inhalation for Stress Eating

Energy-Boosting Peppermint Water

Gentle Detoxifying Lemon Drink

Digestion-Soothing Ginger Oil

Metabolism-Boosting Drink

Calming Bergamot Drink

Anti-Cellulite Bath

Appetite-Suppressant Diffusion

Sandalwood Stomach Rub

Confidence-Boosting Inhalation

Energy-Boosting Foot Rub

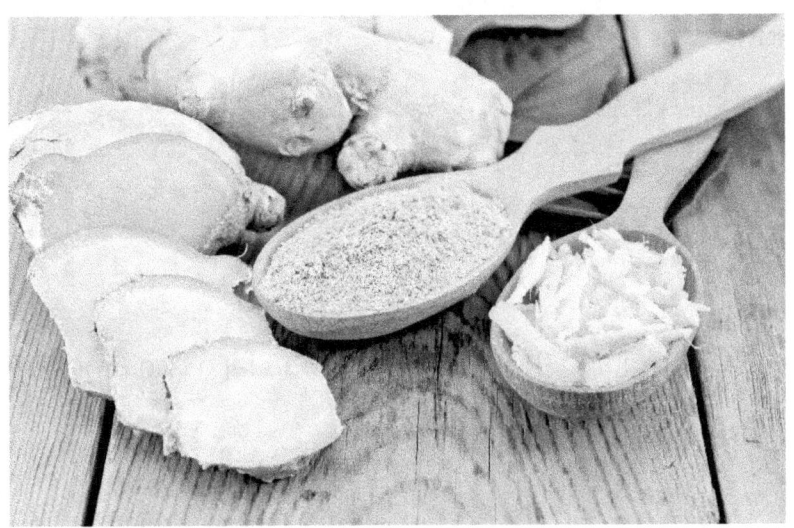

Ingredients:

4 drops lemon essential oil

4 drops ginger essential oil

Instructions:

1. Combine the essential oils in a spoon or small bowl.
2. Rub the oil mixture into the soles of your feet for 5 minutes each to increase energy.

Fat-Blasting Grapefruit Rub

Ingredients:

2 ounces extra-virgin olive oil

5 drops grapefruit essential oil

Instructions:

1. Combine the grapefruit essential oil and the olive oil in a small bowl.
2. Massage the mixture into the skin on places where fat is accumulated.
3. Keep massaging the oils in for about 30 minutes then do not wash it off for at least a few hours.

Cinnamon Drink for Fullness

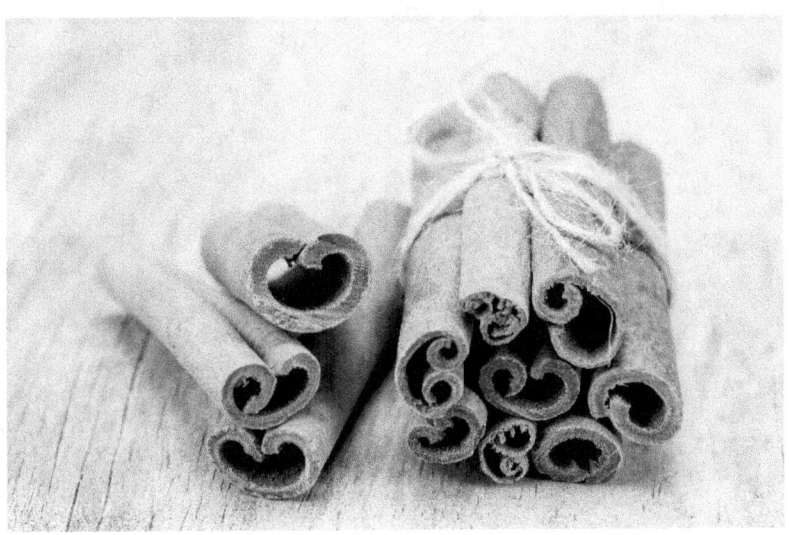

Ingredients:

6 to 8 ounces warm water

1 teaspoon honey

2 to 3 drops cinnamon essential oil

Instructions:

1. Warm the water in a mug using the microwave or a kettle on the stove.
2. Whisk in the honey and cinnamon essential oil.

3. Enjoy the beverage before breakfast in the morning and again before bed to help promote fullness during meals.

Refreshing, Anti-Stress Bath

Ingredients:

Warm water, as needed

2 drops bergamot essential oil

2 drops grapefruit essential oil

Instructions:

1. Draw a warm bath then add the essential oils.
2. Stir the water gently by hand to disperse the oils.
3. Soak in the bath for at least 30 minutes in the morning to reduce stress and refresh yourself.

Lemon Detox Massage

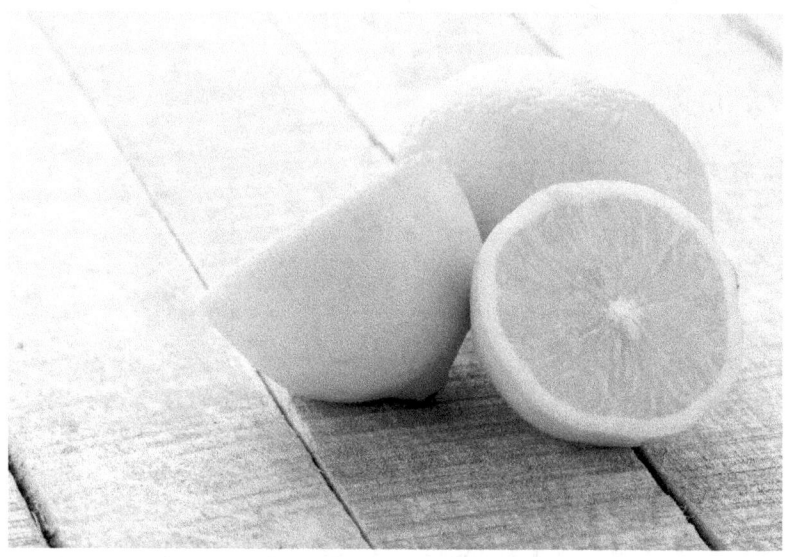

Ingredients:

4 to 6 drops lemon essential oil

Instructions:

1. Massage the oil into areas with heavy cellulite to help eliminate toxins and to encourage release of stored fats.

Pre-Dinner Appetite Suppressant

Ingredients:

2 to 3 drops peppermint essential oil

Instructions:

1. Place a few drops of peppermint essential oil in a diffuser.
2. Inhale the diffused essential oil before eating to reduce your appetite.

Soothing Sandalwood Coconut Milk Beverage

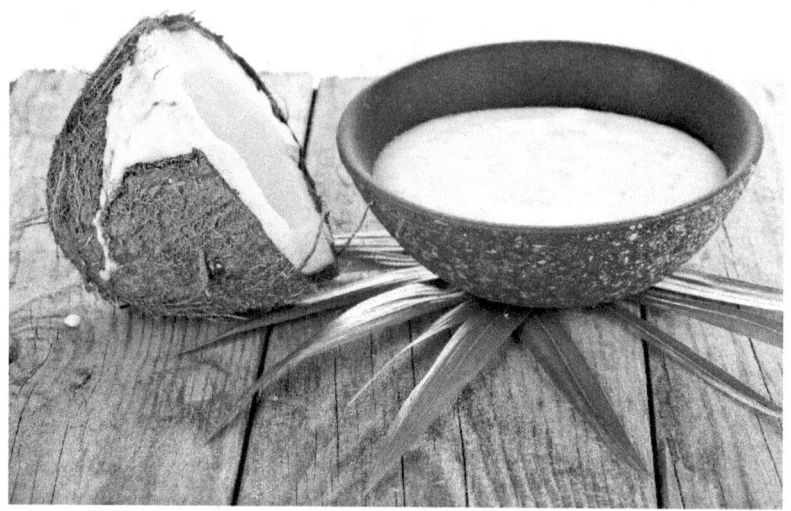

Ingredients:

4 to 6 ounces coconut milk beverage

1 teaspoon honey

1 to 2 drops sandalwood essential oil

Instructions:

1. Warm the coconut milk in a mug in the microwave.
2. Whisk in the honey and sandalwood essential oil.

3. Enjoy the warm drink to calm your mind and body in support of your weight loss efforts.

Craving-Cutting Inhalation

Ingredients:

1 ounce extra-virgin olive oil

5 drops grapefruit essential oil

5 drops sandalwood essential oil

Instructions:

1. Combine the essential oils in a small, dark glass bottle.
2. Swirl the oils to combine.
3. Inhale from the bottle when you feel a craving coming on.

Uplifting Peppermint Rub

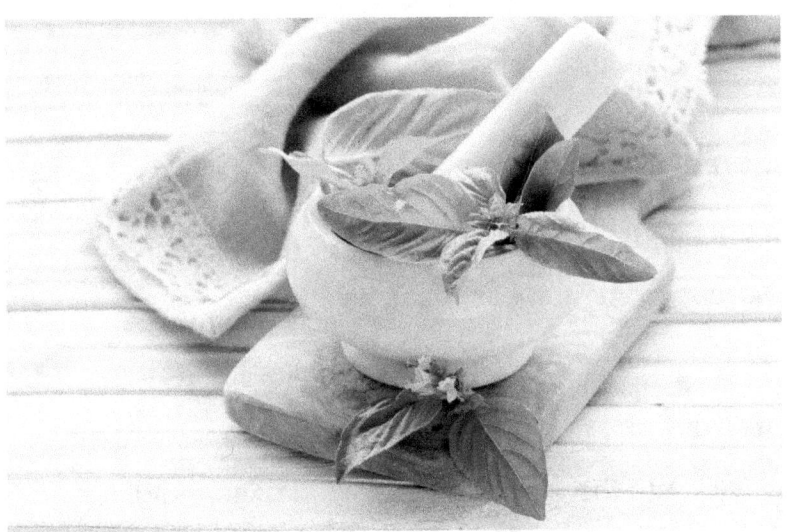

Ingredients:

1 to 2 drops peppermint essential oil

Instructions:

1. Apply the essential oil to the palm of one hand.
2. Rub the oil into the skin over your solar plexus for uplifting and motivation.

Anti-Bloat Grapefruit Drink

Ingredients:

8 ounces filtered water

2 drops grapefruit essential oil

Instructions:

1. Add the grapefruit essential oil to the glass of water.
2. Stir well then drink the entire glass in the morning to flush out toxins that lead to bloating.

Bergamot Craving Suppressant Inhalation

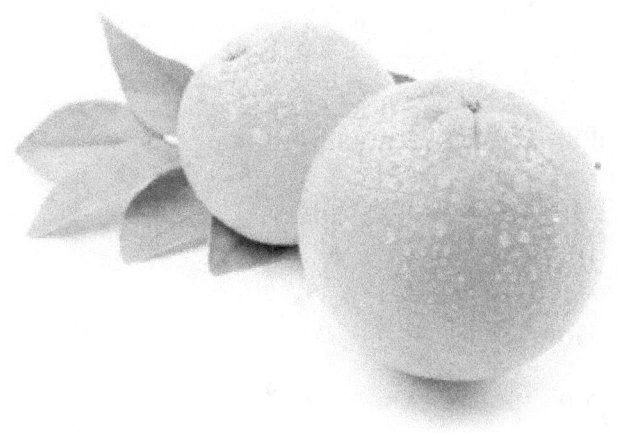

Ingredients:

2 to 3 drops bergamot essential oil

Clean cloth

Instructions:

1. Place a few drops of bergamot essential oil in a clean cloth.
2. Lie down in a comfortable position and drape the cloth over your face.
3. Inhale the essential oil to relieve stress and to suppress cravings.

Appetite-Reducing Grapefruit Inhalation

Ingredients:

1 ounce extra-virgin olive oil

5 drops grapefruit essential oil

3 drops cinnamon essential oil

3 drops sandalwood essential oil

Instructions:

1. Combine the essential oils in a small, dark glass bottle.
2. Swirl the oils to combine.
3. Inhale from the bottle when you feel a craving coming on.

All-Day Weight Loss Drink

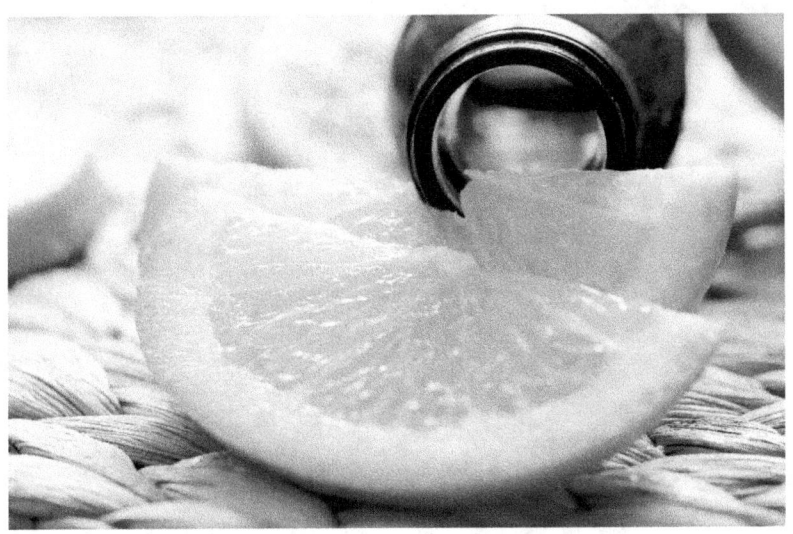

Ingredients:

16 to 24 ounces filtered water

3 drops grapefruit essential oil

1 drop lemon essential oil

1 drop bergamot essential oil

Instructions:

1. Place the water in a large water bottle (with a lid).
2. Add the essential oils and swirl gently to disperse them.

3. Sip on the water throughout the day to suppress your appetite and boost your metabolism.

Soothing Detoxification Bath

Ingredients:

Warm water, as needed

6 drops grapefruit essential oil

6 drops lemon essential oil

6 drops orange essential oil

6 drops ginger essential oil

½ cup apple cider vinegar

Instructions:

1. Draw a warm bath.
2. Add the essential oils and apple cider vinegar and stir gently.
3. Soak in the bath for at least 30 minutes then towel dry to enjoy detoxification benefits.

Appetite-Suppressant Cinnamon Inhalation

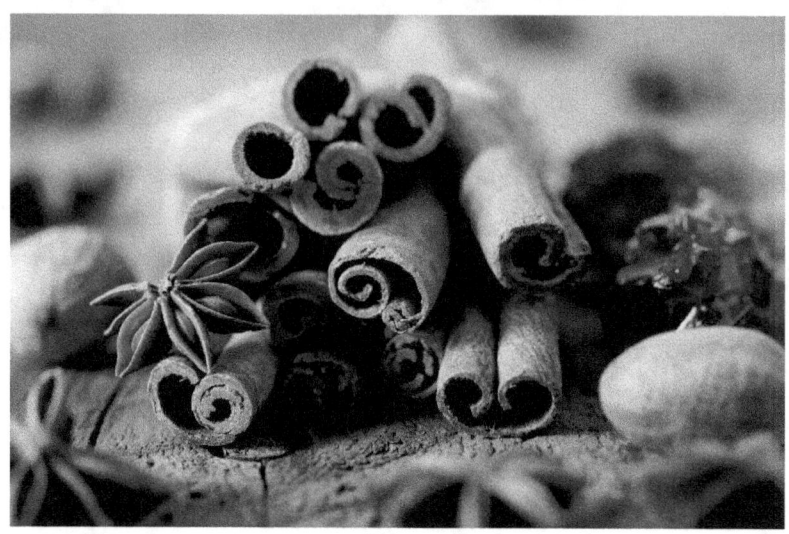

Ingredients:

2 to 3 drops cinnamon essential oil

Instructions:

1. Place a few drops of cinnamon essential oil in a diffuser.
2. Inhale the diffusion before meals to reduce your appetite.

Sandalwood Inhalation for Stress Eating

Ingredients:

3 drops extra-virgin olive oil

3 drops sandalwood essential oil

Instructions:

1. Combine the essential oil and olive oil in a diffuser.
2. Inhale the diffusion to combat stress eating and cravings.

Energy-Boosting Peppermint Water

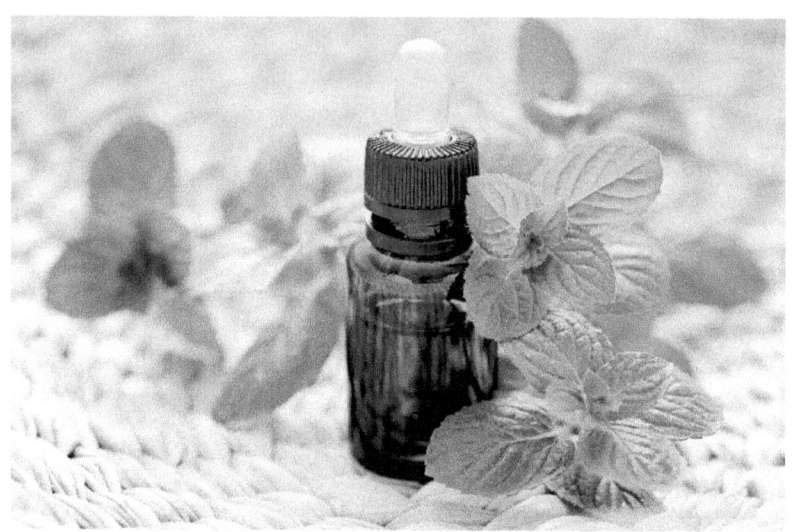

Ingredients:

8 ounces filtered water

2 to 3 drops peppermint essential oil

Instructions:

1. Add the peppermint essential oil to a glass of filtered water.
2. Stir well then drink the whole glass before working out to boost your energy.
3. You can also enjoy this drink before a meal to reduce your appetite.

Gentle Detoxifying Lemon Drink

Ingredients:

8 ounces filtered water

2 drops lemon essential oil

Instructions:

1. Add the lemon essential oil to the water and stir well.
2. Drink the entire glass in the morning before breakfast to encourage gentle detoxification throughout the day.

Digestion-Soothing Ginger Oil

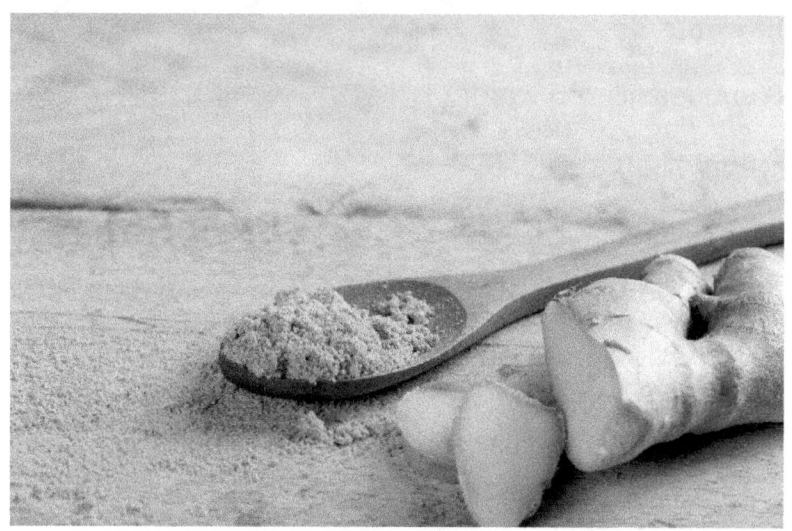

Ingredients:

1 to 2 drops ginger essential oil

1 drop cinnamon essential oil

Instructions:

1. Rub the essential oils into the skin over your abdomen.
2. Massage the abdomen for at least 15 minutes, moving your hands in the direction of digestion to relieve digestive issues.

Metabolism-Boosting Drink

Ingredients:

8 ounces filtered water

2 drops ginger essential oil

1 to 2 drops lemon essential oil

Instructions:

1. Add the essential oils to a glass of filtered water.
2. Stir well then drink the whole glass in the morning to boost your metabolism.

Calming Bergamot Drink

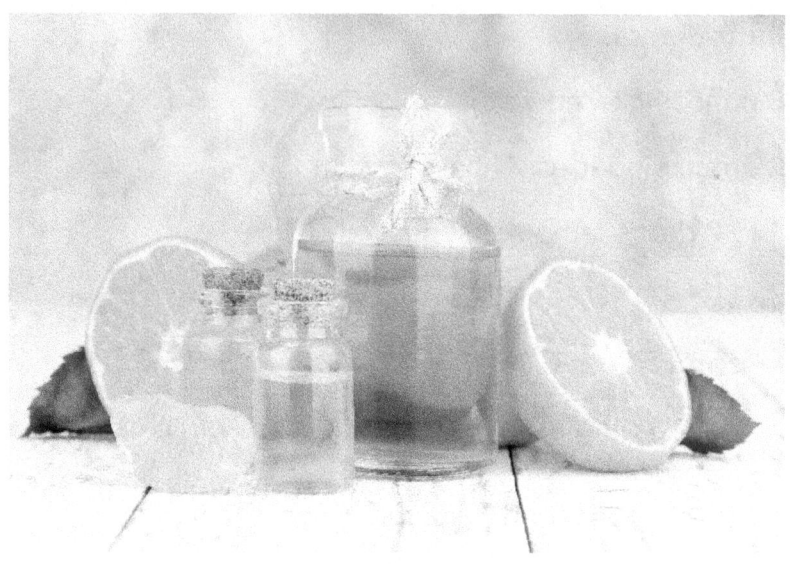

Ingredients:

4 to 6 ounces coconut milk beverage

1 teaspoon honey

1 to 2 drops bergamot essential oil

Instructions:

1. Warm the coconut milk in a mug in the microwave.
2. Whisk in the honey and bergamot essential oil.

3. Enjoy the warm drink to calm your mind and body in support of your weight loss efforts.

Anti-Cellulite Bath

Ingredients:

Warm water, as needed

5 drops grapefruit essential oil

5 drips ginger essential oil

5 drops orange essential oil

5 drops sandalwood essential oil

Instructions:

1. Draw a warm bath.
2. Add the essential oils and stir the water gently to disperse them.
3. Soak in the bath for at least 30 minutes to reduce the appearance of cellulite.
4. Towel dry after the bath.

Appetite-Suppressant Diffusion

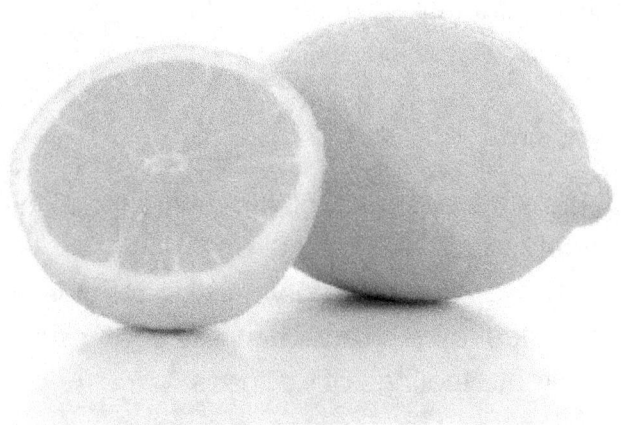

Ingredients:

2 to 3 drops lemon essential oil

Instructions:

1. Place a few drops of lemon essential oil in a diffuser.
2. Inhale the diffusion before meals to reduce your appetite.

Sandalwood Stomach Rub

Ingredients:

3 to 4 drops sandalwood essential oil

Instructions:

1. Apply the essential oil directly to the skin over your stomach.
2. Massage the oils into your skin for at least 15 minutes to help reduce stress eating and to promote feelings of wellness.

Confidence-Boosting Inhalation

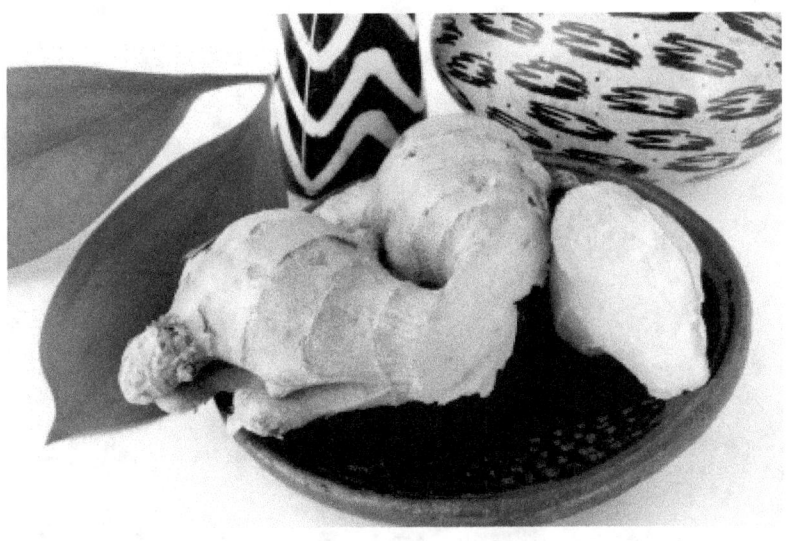

Ingredients:

2 drops ginger essential oil

2 drops cinnamon essential oil

Instructions:

1. Place the essential oils in a diffuser.
2. Inhale the diffusion to boost your confidence and combat stress eating.

Conclusion

If you feel as though you have been struggling to lose weight and nothing you try actually works, this is the perfect book for you. Essential oils are all-natural, derived from a variety of different plants, and they can provide myriad health benefits related to weight loss. Certain essential oils can help to curb your cravings, reduce your appetite, or detoxify your body. If you are ready to jump-start your weight loss efforts, select a recipe from this book and give it a go!

www.ingramcontent.com/pod-product-compliance
Lightning Source LLC
Chambersburg PA
CBHW060345290526
45791CB00004B/1537